The 30-Day Digital Detox Challenge

Reclaim Your Time, Focus, and Happiness

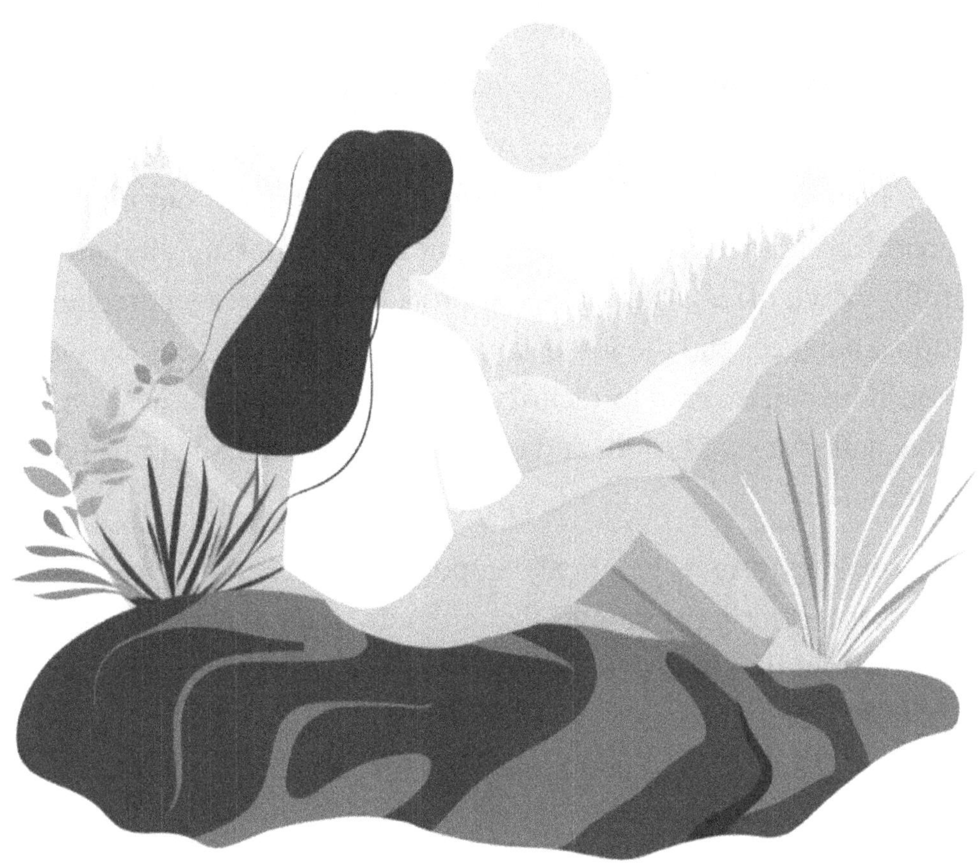

By

Aliyu Aminu Ahmed

Foreword

In a world that never stops buzzing, where our lives are increasingly intertwined with the digital, it's easy to feel overwhelmed, disconnected, and even lost in the constant stream of notifications and virtual engagements. Technology has revolutionized how we live and work, offering immense benefits, but it has also introduced new challenges that can erode our sense of well-being, productivity, and even our personal relationships.

In The 30-Day Digital Detox Challenge, Aliyu Aminu Ahmed provides an insightful, timely guide to help us navigate the complexities of our digital lives. This book is not about rejecting technology, but about understanding how to use it more mindfully. Aliyu offers a structured approach to help readers reclaim their focus, emotional balance, and the joy of living fully in the present. By taking the challenge, you'll be empowered to identify your digital habits, assess their impact on your mental and physical health, and ultimately, re-establish control over your time and attention.

What sets this book apart is its practical, supportive nature. Aliyu walks with you through the process, offering strategies that are both achievable and sustainable. Whether you're struggling with social media overuse, constant work emails, or just looking for a way to reconnect with your offline self, The 30-Day Digital Detox Challenge is a tool that will help you achieve lasting change.

In a world where digital distractions can pull us away from the things that matter most, this book serves as a refreshing call to reclaim balance. Aliyu's expertise and thoughtful guidance will lead you toward a healthier, more intentional relationship with technology. I encourage you to embrace this challenge—not as a break from technology, but as a step toward living a more purposeful and mindful life.

Ruqayya Muhammad

About the Book

The 30-Day Digital Detox Challenge by Aliyu Aminu Ahmed is a comprehensive guide designed to help individuals break free from the overwhelming grip of technology and restore balance in their lives. In this fast-paced digital era, where screens dominate nearly every aspect of our daily routines, this book offers a structured approach to creating healthier habits and more intentional digital use. Through a series of practical, step-by-step activities spread over 30 days, readers are encouraged to reflect on their relationship with technology, identify triggers for overuse, and implement meaningful changes. The challenge is not about cutting off technology altogether, but about reclaiming time, focus, and mental clarity.

Aliyu's insightful approach offers practical tips for managing screen time, dealing with digital addiction, and developing a more mindful relationship with technology. From setting tech-free zones in your home to reintroducing devices mindfully after the detox, each chapter empowers readers to replace mindless scrolling with enriching activities that foster well-being, creativity, and deeper connections with others. Whether you're seeking to reduce stress, improve productivity, or simply disconnect from the constant noise of the digital world, The 30-Day Digital Detox Challenge provides the tools and inspiration to make lasting, positive changes in your life.

Contents

Introduction

The 30-Day Digital Detox Challenge

In today's fast-paced, hyper-connected world, our lives are increasingly intertwined with technology. While the digital landscape offers remarkable conveniences and opportunities, it also presents challenges that can leave us feeling overwhelmed, distracted, and disconnected from what truly matters.

The constant barrage of notifications, social media updates, and digital distractions can lead to an unhealthy relationship with our devices, often resulting in stress, anxiety, and a diminished sense of well-being.

Welcome to the 30-Day Digital Detox Challenge, a transformative journey designed to help you reclaim your time, focus, and happiness. This challenge is not just about unplugging from your devices; it's about reconnecting with yourself, your loved ones, and the world around you. Over the next month, you will embark on a structured and supportive detox process that encourages you to evaluate your digital habits, identify triggers, and develop healthier routines.

Why a Digital Detox?

The importance of a digital detox cannot be overstated. Research shows that excessive screen time can lead to a range of negative effects, including decreased productivity, impaired sleep, and increased feelings of loneliness and isolation. By taking a step back from technology, you can create space for self-reflection, personal growth, and meaningful connections.

This challenge is designed for anyone who feels overwhelmed by their digital life—whether you're a busy professional, a student, a parent, or simply someone looking to find balance in a tech-saturated world. The 30-Day Digital Detox Challenge offers practical strategies, engaging activities, and supportive resources to guide you through this transformative experience.

What to Expect

Throughout this book, you will find a step-by-step roadmap to help you navigate your digital detox journey. Each week will focus on different aspects of your relationship with technology, providing you with the tools and insights needed to make lasting changes. You will learn how to set achievable goals, identify your digital triggers, and replace screen time with enriching activities that promote well-being without impacting on your regular job! I promise.

As you progress through the challenge, you'll discover the profound benefits of unplugging: improved focus, enhanced creativity, deeper relationships, and a renewed sense of joy in everyday life. You will also have the opportunity to reflect on your experiences, celebrate your successes, and share your journey with others, creating a sense of community and accountability.

Embrace the Challenge

Are you ready to take the plunge? Embrace the 30-Day Digital Detox Challenge as an opportunity to break free from the confines of your screen and rediscover what it means to live fully in the moment. Let this journey inspire you to cultivate a healthier relationship with technology, one that enhances your life rather than detracts from it.

Join me as we embark on this exciting adventure together. Let's reclaim our time, focus, and happiness—one day at a time.

Chapter 1

Understanding the Digital Dilemma

The Impact of Technology on Daily Life

In the contemporary landscape, technology permeates every aspect of our daily lives. From the moment we wake up to the sound of our smartphones to the last scroll through social media before bed, digital devices have become integral to our routines. According to a Pew Research Center survey, 28% of global adults report being online "almost constantly," a significant increase from previous years (Pew Research Center, 2021). This constant connectivity offers undeniable advantages, such as instant access to information, enhanced communication, and the convenience of online services. However, it also presents a paradox: while technology can improve our lives, it can also lead to detrimental effects on our mental and physical well-being.

The omnipresence of digital devices has altered how we interact with the world. Work-life boundaries have blurred, with many individuals feeling the pressure to remain connected to their jobs outside of traditional hours (Gajendran & Harrison, 2007). Social interactions have shifted from face-to-face conversations to digital exchanges, often leading to feelings of isolation and disconnection (Primack et al., 2017). The impact of technology on daily life is profound, affecting not only our productivity but also our emotional health and interpersonal relationships.

Recognizing Digital Addiction

As technology continues to evolve, so too does the phenomenon of digital addiction. Digital addiction, often referred to as technology addiction or internet addiction, is characterized by a compulsive and excessive use of digital devices that interferes with daily functioning. This addiction is not formally recognized in the Diagnostic and Statistical Manual of Mental Disorders (DSM-5), yet it is increasingly acknowledged by mental health professionals as a significant concern in modern society (American Psychological Association, 2017).

Digital addiction manifests in various forms, including social media addiction, gaming addiction, and compulsive internet browsing. Individuals may find themselves spending hours online, neglecting responsibilities, and experiencing withdrawal symptoms when unable to access their devices (Kuss & Griffiths, 2017). The compulsive nature of digital addiction can lead to a cycle of dependence, where the individual feels compelled to engage with technology despite negative consequences.

Recognizing the signs of digital addiction is crucial for intervention and recovery. Key indicators include:

- **Preoccupation with Technology:** Constantly thinking about online activities or anticipating the next time one will be online (American Psychological Association, 2017).
- **Loss of Control:** Unsuccessful attempts to cut back on device use, often leading to extended periods of online activity (Kuss & Griffiths, 2017).
- **Neglect of Responsibilities:** Ignoring work, school, or personal obligations in favor of online engagement (American Psychological Association, 2017).
- **Emotional Distress:** Experiencing irritability, anxiety, or depression when unable to use digital devices (Kuss & Griffiths, 2017).

Symptoms of Overuse: Mental and Physical Effects

The consequences of digital addiction extend beyond mere inconvenience; they can significantly impact both mental and physical health. Research indicates that excessive screen time is linked to a variety of mental health issues, including anxiety, depression, and sleep disorders (Twenge, 2019). The World Health Organization has recognized the detrimental effects of excessive digital technology use, particularly in terms of sleep disturbances and emotional well-being (World Health Organization, 2019).

Mental Effects

The mental effects are as follows:

- **Anxiety and Depression:** Prolonged exposure to digital devices can lead to increased feelings of anxiety and depression. The constant comparison to others on social media, coupled with the pressure to maintain an online presence, can exacerbate feelings of inadequacy and isolation (Twenge, 2019).

- **Cognitive Impairment:** Excessive screen time can impair cognitive functions, including attention span, memory, and decision-making abilities. The brain's reward system becomes overstimulated, leading to difficulties in focusing on tasks that do not provide immediate gratification (Uncapher & Wagner, 2018).
- **Social Isolation:** While technology facilitates communication, it can also lead to social isolation. Individuals may prioritize online interactions over in-person relationships, resulting in a lack of meaningful connections and support (Primack et al., 2017).

Physical Effects

There are also physical effects such as:

- **Sleep Disorders:** The blue light emitted by screens can disrupt circadian rhythms, leading to difficulties in falling asleep and maintaining restful sleep. Insomnia and other sleep disorders are common among those who engage in excessive screen time, further exacerbating mental health issues (Fossum et al., 2014).
- **Physical Health Issues:** Prolonged periods of inactivity associated with excessive device use can lead to a range of physical health problems, including obesity, cardiovascular issues, and musculoskeletal disorders. Conditions such as carpal tunnel syndrome, eye strain, and poor posture are also prevalent among individuals who spend significant time on digital devices (Straker et al., 2018).
- **Addictive Behaviors:** Digital addiction can lead to other unhealthy behaviors, such as poor eating habits, lack of physical activity, and neglect of self-care routines. This cycle of addiction can create a negative feedback loop, where the individual turns to technology as a coping mechanism for stress, further entrenching their dependence (Kuss & Griffiths, 2017).

Overall, understanding the digital dilemma is the first step toward addressing the challenges posed by technology in our lives. By recognizing the impact of technology on daily life, acknowledging the signs of digital addiction, and being aware of the mental and physical symptoms of overuse, individuals can begin to take proactive steps toward a healthier relationship with their devices. The 30-Day Digital Detox Challenge offers a structured approach to help navigate these issues, empowering individuals to reclaim their time, focus, and happiness in an increasingly digital world.

References

- American Psychological Association. (2017). Internet gaming disorder. https://www.apa.org/topics/internet-gaming-disorder
- Fossum, I. N., Nordnes, L. T., Storemark, S. S., Bjorvatn, B., & Pallesen, S. (2014). The association between use of electronic media in bed before going to sleep and insomnia symptoms, daytime sleepiness, morningness, and chronotype. Behavioral Sleep Medicine, 12(5), 343-357. https://doi.org/10.1080/15402002.2013.819468
- Gajendran, R. S., & Harrison, D. A. (2007). The good, the bad, and the unknown about telecommuting: Meta-analysis of psychological mediators and individual consequences. Journal of Applied Psychology, 92(6), 1524-1541. https://doi.org/10.1037/0021-9010.92.6.1524
- Kuss, D. J., & Griffiths, M. D. (2017). Social networking sites and addiction: Ten lessons learned. International Journal of Environmental Research and Public Health, 14(3), 311. https://doi.org/10.3390/ijerph14030311
- Pew Research Center. (2021). About a quarter of U.S. adults say they are 'almost constantly' online. https://www.pewresearch.org/fact-tank/2021/03/26/about-a-quarter-of-u-s-adults-say-they-are-almost-constantly-online/
- Primack, B. A., Shensa, A., Sidani, J. E., Whaite, E. O., Lin, L. Y., Rosen, D., Colditz, J. B., Radovic, A., & Miller, E. (2017). Social media use and perceived social isolation among young adults in the U.S. American Journal of Preventive Medicine, 53(1), 1-8. https://doi.org/10.1016/j.amepre.2017.01.010
- Straker, L., Zabatiero, J., Danby, S., Thorpe, K., & Edwards, S. (2018). Conflicting guidelines on young children's screen time and use of digital

technology create policy and practice dilemmas. The Journal of Pediatrics, 202, 300-303. https://doi.org/10.1016/j.jpeds.2018.07.019

- Twenge, J. M. (2019). More time on technology, less time talking? Increases in impersonal communication and decreases in face-to-face communication in the United States in the 21st century. Review of General Psychology, 23(2), 223-242. https://doi.org/10.1177/1089268019846208
- Uncapher, M. R., & Wagner, A. D. (2018). Minds and brains of media multitaskers: Current findings and future directions. Proceedings of the National Academy of Sciences, 115(40), 9889-9896. https://doi.org/10.1073/pnas.1611612115
- World Health Organization. (2019). Guidelines on physical activity, sedentary behaviour and sleep for children under 5 years of age. https://apps.who.int/iris/bitstream/handle/10665/311664/9789241550536-eng.pdf

Chapter 2

Preparing for the 30-Day Challenge

Setting Achievable Goals for Your Digital Detox

Before embarking on your 30-Day Digital Detox Challenge, it's crucial to set clear and achievable goals that align with your motivations for unplugging.

According to Locke and Latham's goal-setting theory, specific and challenging goals lead to higher performance and satisfaction (Locke & Latham, 2002). By establishing well-defined objectives, you provide yourself with a roadmap for success and a means to measure your progress throughout the detox.

When setting your goals, consider the specific areas of your digital life you want to address. Do you aim to reduce social media usage, limit email checking, or completely abstain from certain devices? Be as specific as possible in quantifying your goals, such as setting a daily time limit for social media or committing to checking emails only during designated work hours. Additionally, ensure that your goals are realistic and attainable to maintain motivation and avoid discouragement.

It's also beneficial to set both short-term and long-term goals for your digital detox. Short-term goals, such as completing a 24-hour device-free period or engaging in a specific number of offline activities per day, provide a sense of immediate accomplishment and help you build momentum. Long-term goals, such as developing healthier digital habits or experiencing improved mental well-being, give you a broader perspective on the potential benefits of your detox and keep you focused on the bigger picture.

Creating a Supportive Environment for Success

Preparing a supportive environment is crucial for the success of your 30-Day Digital Detox Challenge. By minimizing temptations and creating physical and mental spaces conducive to unplugging, you increase your chances of sticking to your goals and experiencing the full benefits of your detox.

One effective strategy is to designate device-free zones in your home, such as the bedroom or dining area, where you refrain from using digital devices (Arootah, 2022). This helps create a sense of sanctuary and encourages you to be present in the moment, fostering deeper connections with loved ones and promoting better sleep hygiene.

Additionally, consider involving your family and friends in your digital detox journey. Encourage them to support your goals and participate in offline activities together, such as board game nights, outdoor adventures, or tech-free social gatherings (Edufun Technik, 2022). Having a supportive network can provide accountability, motivation, and a sense of community throughout your detox experience.

Identifying Your Unique Triggers and Patterns

To effectively manage your digital habits during the 30-Day Digital Detox Challenge, it's essential to identify your unique triggers and patterns of technology use. By understanding the situations, emotions, and behaviors that drive your excessive screen time, you can develop strategies to mitigate these factors and maintain a healthier relationship with technology.

Begin by tracking your digital usage over a few days, noting when and why you engage with your devices. Are there specific times of day when you find yourself mindlessly scrolling? Do certain emotions, such as boredom or stress, lead you to seek refuge in your smartphone? Identifying these patterns can help you anticipate potential challenges and plan accordingly.

Next, consider the specific apps, websites, or devices that tend to consume the most of your time and attention. Social media platforms, email, and instant messaging are common culprits, often providing a constant stream of stimulation and a sense of FOMO (fear of missing out) (Kuss & Griffiths, 2017). By being aware of your most significant digital temptations, you can take proactive steps to limit or avoid them during your detox.

Remember, everyone's relationship with technology is unique, shaped by individual circumstances, preferences, and habits. Embrace the process of self-discovery during this preparatory phase, and be open to adjusting your strategies as you progress through the 30-Day Digital Detox Challenge.

Overall, preparing for the 30-Day Digital Detox Challenge involves setting achievable goals, creating a supportive environment, and identifying your unique triggers and patterns. By taking these proactive steps, you lay the foundation for a successful detox experience and increase your chances of developing healthier digital habits that last long after the challenge is complete. Embrace this preparatory phase as an opportunity to gain clarity, build momentum, and embark on your journey to reclaim your time, focus, and happiness in a technology-driven world.

References

Arootah. (2022). 7 ways to do a successful digital detox this holiday season. https://arootah.com/blog/health-and-wellbeing/how-to-do-a-successful-digital-detox/

Edufun Technik. (2022). 9 clever hacks for peaceful device detox with kids. https://edufuntechnik.com/9-clever-hacks-for-peaceful-device-detox-with-kids/

Kuss, D. J., & Griffiths, M. D. (2017). Social networking sites and addiction: Ten lessons learned. International Journal of Environmental Research and Public Health, 14(3), 311. https://doi.org/10.3390/ijerph14030311

Locke, E. A., & Latham, G. P. (2002). Building a practically useful theory of goal setting and task motivation: A 35-year odyssey. American Psychologist, 57(9), 705-717. https://doi.org/10.1037/0003-066X.57.9.705

Chapter 3

Tackling the Detox Process

Embarking on a digital detox is a significant step toward reclaiming your time, focus, and happiness. However, the approach you choose to take during this process can greatly influence your success. In this chapter, we will explore two primary methods for tackling your detox: going "cold turkey" versus gradual reduction. Additionally, we will discuss engaging in activities to replace screen time and the importance of reconnecting with nature and community.

Choosing Your Approach: Cold Turkey or Gradual Reduction

When it comes to digital detoxing, individuals often find themselves choosing between two distinct approaches: going "cold turkey" or gradually reducing their screen time. Each method has its own advantages and challenges, and the best choice depends on your personal preferences, habits, and goals.

The Cold Turkey Approach

The cold turkey method involves completely eliminating or significantly reducing your digital device usage all at once. This approach can be particularly effective for individuals who feel overwhelmed by their technology use and want to make a swift change. By removing devices from your daily routine entirely, you can create a clear boundary that allows for a fresh start.

Advantages:

- **Immediate Impact:** A sudden break from technology can lead to rapid changes in mental clarity, productivity, and emotional well-being.
- **Clear Boundaries:** Going cold turkey establishes a definitive cutoff point, making it easier to avoid temptation and distractions.

Challenges:

- **Withdrawal Symptoms:** Some individuals may experience feelings of anxiety, irritability, or restlessness when suddenly disconnected from their devices (Kuss & Griffiths, 2017).
- **Social Pressure:** The cold turkey method may lead to feelings of isolation if friends and family are still engaged in digital activities.

Gradual Reduction Approach

The gradual reduction method involves slowly decreasing your screen time over a set period. This approach allows for a more manageable transition, as you can gradually replace digital activities with offline alternatives.

- **Smoother Transition:** Gradually reducing screen time can help mitigate withdrawal symptoms and make the process feel less daunting.
- **Increased Awareness:** This method encourages mindfulness about your technology use, helping you identify specific habits and triggers.

Challenges:

- **Potential for Slipping:** Without a firm commitment to reducing screen time, some individuals may find it easy to revert to old habits (Rosen et al., 2014).
- Less Immediate Change: The gradual approach may take longer to yield noticeable benefits compared to a cold turkey method.

Ultimately, the choice between cold turkey and gradual reduction depends on your personal comfort level and the specific goals you wish to achieve during your digital detox. Consider experimenting with both methods to see which resonates best with you.

Engaging in Activities to Replace Screen Time

One of the most effective strategies for a successful digital detox is to engage in alternative activities that replace the time previously spent on screens. By filling your schedule with enriching offline experiences, you can redirect your focus and energy toward activities that promote well-being and personal growth.

1. Explore Hobbies and Interests

Rediscovering hobbies that you may have neglected due to excessive screen time can be a fulfilling way to spend your time. Whether it's painting, gardening, cooking, or playing a musical instrument, engaging in creative pursuits can provide a sense of accomplishment and joy (Kuss & Griffiths, 2017).

2. Physical Activity

Incorporating physical activity into your daily routine can have profound benefits for both mental and physical health. Consider activities such as walking, jogging, yoga, or joining a local sports team. Exercise has been shown to reduce symptoms of anxiety and depression, enhance mood, and improve overall well-being (Craft & Perna, 2004).

3. Reading and Learning

Use your newfound free time to read books, articles, or engage in online courses that pique your interest. Reading not only stimulates the mind but also enhances empathy and understanding (Mar et al., 2006). Consider joining a book club to foster social connections while enjoying literature.

4. Socializing Offline

Make a conscious effort to reconnect with friends and family in person. Organize gatherings, game nights, or outdoor activities that encourage face-to-face interactions. Building and maintaining meaningful relationships can significantly enhance your emotional well-being (Holt-Lunstad et al., 2010).

Reconnecting with Nature and Community

In addition to engaging in alternative activities, reconnecting with nature and your local community can be a powerful aspect of your digital detox journey. Nature has been shown to have restorative effects on mental health, reducing stress and enhancing overall well-being (Kaplan & Kaplan, 1989).

1. Spend Time Outdoors

Make it a priority to spend time outdoors, whether through hiking, biking, or simply taking walks in your local park. Nature exposure has been linked to improved mood, reduced anxiety, and increased feelings of connectedness (Barton

& Pretty, 2010). Consider scheduling regular outings to immerse yourself in natural surroundings.

2. Volunteer in Your Community

Engaging in community service or volunteer work can provide a sense of purpose and fulfillment while fostering connections with others. Look for local organizations or initiatives that align with your interests and values. Volunteering not only benefits the community but also enhances your own well-being by promoting feelings of gratitude and empathy (Post, 2005).

3. Join Local Groups or Clubs

Participating in local clubs or groups that align with your interests can help you build connections and expand your social network. Whether it's a hiking club, a gardening group, or a community class, joining others who share your passions can lead to meaningful relationships and experiences.

Overall, tackling the detox process involves choosing the right approach, engaging in alternative activities, and reconnecting with nature and community. By thoughtfully navigating these aspects of your digital detox, you can create a fulfilling and enriching experience that allows you to reclaim your time, focus, and happiness. Embrace this journey as an opportunity for self-discovery and growth, and enjoy the benefits of a more balanced relationship with technology.

References

Barton, J., & Pretty, J. (2010). What is the best dose of nature and green exercise for improving mental health? A multi-study analysis. Environmental Science & Technology, 44(10), 3947-3955.

Craft, L. L., & Perna, F. M. (2004). The benefits of exercise for the clinically depressed. Primary Care Companion to The Journal of Clinical Psychiatry, 6(3), 104-111. https://doi.org/10.4088/PCC.v06n0301

Kaplan, R., & Kaplan, S. (1989). The experience of nature: A psychological perspective. Cambridge University Press.

Kuss, D. J., & Griffiths, M. D. (2017). Social networking sites and addiction: Ten lessons learned. International Journal of Environmental Research and Public Health, 14(3), 311. https://doi.org/10.3390/ijerph14030311

Mar, R. A., Oatley, K., Hirsh, J., dela Paz, J., & Peterson, J. B. (2006). Book reading, empathy, and social ability. Scientific Studies of Reading, 10(4), 327-352. https://doi.org/10.1207/s1532799xssr1004_2

Post, S. G. (2005). Altruism, happiness, and health: It's good to be good. International Journal of Behavioral Medicine, 12(2), 66-77. https://doi.org/10.1207/s15327558ijbm1202_1

Rosen, L. D., Lim, AF., Carrier, LM., & Cheever, NA. (2014). An empirical examination of the educational impact of cell phone use in the classroom. Computers & Education, 69, 69-75. https://doi.org/10.1016/j.compedu.2013.12.001

Chapter 4

Developing Healthy Digital Habits

In the journey toward reclaiming your time, focus, and happiness, developing healthy digital habits is essential. This chapter will guide you through establishing routines for mindful technology use, reintroducing technology mindfully after your detox, and implementing long-term strategies for maintaining balance in your digital life.

Establishing Routines for Mindful Technology Use

Mindful technology use involves being intentional and aware of how and why you engage with digital devices. According to the definition provided by the Ohio State University, mindful technology use is knowing what you are doing with technology and why you are doing it (Ohio State University, n.d.). This awareness is crucial in preventing mindless scrolling and compulsive checking of notifications.

To establish routines for mindful technology use, consider the following strategies:

- **Set Boundaries:** Create specific times during the day dedicated to technology use. For example, designate certain hours for checking emails or social media and stick to these times. Outside of these periods, keep your devices out of sight to resist temptation (Dwase, 2022).
- **Create Tech-Free Zones:** Designate areas in your home where technology is not allowed, such as the dining room or bedroom. This encourages more

meaningful interactions with family and friends and promotes better sleep hygiene by reducing blue light exposure before bedtime (Zario, n.d.).

- **Track Your Screen Time:** Utilize built-in features on your devices, such as Apple's Screen Time or Android's Digital Wellbeing tools, to monitor your usage patterns. This awareness can help you identify areas where you may need to cut back (Tech.gov.sg, 2021).
- **Mindful Breaks:** Incorporate regular breaks from technology throughout your day. During these breaks, practice mindfulness techniques such as deep breathing or stretching to recharge your mind and body (Dwase, 2022).

Reintroducing Technology Mindfully After the Challenge

After completing your digital detox, it is essential to reintroduce technology mindfully. This phase is crucial for ensuring that the positive changes you experienced during the detox are maintained in the long run. Here are some strategies for a mindful reintroduction:

- **Evaluate Your Needs:** Reflect on your experiences during the detox. Consider which digital activities added value to your life and which ones felt burdensome. Use this reflection to guide your choices as you reintroduce technology (Arootah, 2022).
- **Gradual Reintroduction:** Instead of diving back into full technology use, gradually reintroduce apps and devices into your routine. Start with essential tools for work or communication, and monitor how they affect your well-being (Zario, n.d.).
- **Set New Limits:** Establish new limits for technology use based on your reflections from the detox. For instance, if social media was a significant source of distraction, consider limiting your usage to specific times of day or using apps that restrict access (Kuss & Griffiths, 2017).
- **Prioritize Quality Over Quantity:** Focus on engaging with technology that enhances your life. Choose apps and platforms that promote well-being,

such as meditation or fitness apps, rather than those that contribute to mindless scrolling (Tech.gov.sg, 2021).

Long-Term Strategies for Maintaining Balance

To ensure that you maintain a healthy relationship with technology in the long term, consider implementing the following strategies:

- **Regular Digital Detoxes:** Incorporate regular digital detoxes into your routine, whether it's a weekly tech-free day or an annual retreat. These breaks can help reset your relationship with technology and reinforce the habits you've developed (Zario, n.d.).
- **Engage in Offline Activities:** Continuously prioritize offline activities that promote well-being, such as exercise, reading, or spending time with loved ones. Engaging in these activities can help reduce reliance on digital devices for fulfillment (Dwase, 2022).
- **Cultivate a Mindful Mindset:** Embrace a mindset of mindfulness in your daily life. Regularly check in with yourself to assess how technology is impacting your mood and productivity. If you notice negative effects, adjust your habits accordingly (Kuss & Griffiths, 2017).
- **Seek Support:** Share your goals and experiences with friends and family. Having a support system can provide accountability and encouragement as you navigate your digital habits (Arootah, 2022).

Overall, developing healthy digital habits is an ongoing process that requires intention and awareness. By establishing routines for mindful technology use, reintroducing technology thoughtfully after your detox, and implementing long-term strategies for maintaining balance, you can create a fulfilling and enriching relationship with technology. Embrace this journey as an opportunity for growth and self-discovery, and enjoy the benefits of a more balanced digital life.

References

- Arootah. (2022). 7 ways to do a successful digital detox this holiday season. https://arootah.com/blog/health-and-wellbeing/how-to-do-a-successful-digital-detox/
- Dwase, M. (2022). How to incorporate technology into your life in a healthy way. LinkedIn. https://www.linkedin.com/pulse/mindful-technology-use-how-incorporate-your-life-way-mary-dwase
- Kuss, D. J., & Griffiths, M. D. (2017). Social networking sites and addiction: Ten lessons learned. International Journal of Environmental Research and Public Health, 14(3), 311. https://doi.org/10.3390/ijerph14030311
- Ohio State University. (n.d.). Mindful technology use. https://it.osu.edu/learner-technology-handbook/ch4/mindful-technology-use
- Tech.gov.sg. (2021). International Self Care Day: Tips for wellness through mindful tech use. https://www.tech.gov.sg/media/technews/international-self-care-day/
- Zario. (n.d.). Prioritizing digital wellbeing: A guide to mindful technology use. https://www.meetzario.com/post/prioritizing-digital-wellbeing-a-guide-to-mindful-technology-use

Chapter 5

Reflecting on Your Journey

As you near the conclusion of your 30-Day Digital Detox Challenge, it's essential to take the time to reflect on your journey. This chapter will guide you through celebrating your progress and achievements, as well as sharing your experiences with others to inspire change. Reflecting on your journey not only reinforces the positive changes you've made but also helps you solidify the lessons learned and the habits developed during this transformative process.

Celebrating Your Progress and Achievements

Reflecting on your accomplishments is a crucial aspect of personal growth. Celebrating your progress during the digital detox can enhance your motivation and commitment to maintaining healthy digital habits in the future. Here are some ways to effectively celebrate your achievements:

- **Keep a Journal:** Throughout your detox, maintain a journal to document your experiences, thoughts, and feelings. Reflect on how your relationship with technology has changed and note specific instances where you felt more present or engaged in offline activities. At the end of the challenge, review your entries and acknowledge the growth you've experienced (Davis, 2020).
- **Set Milestones:** Identify specific milestones you achieved during the detox, such as completing a week without social media or spending more time outdoors. Celebrate these milestones by treating yourself to something special, whether it's a favorite meal, a day out, or a small gift that

symbolizes your commitment to a healthier relationship with technology (Zario, n.d.).

- **Create a Visual Representation:** Use visual aids to represent your progress, such as a chart or a vision board. Include images, quotes, or symbols that resonate with your journey. Display this visual representation in a prominent place as a reminder of your achievements and the positive changes you've made (Davis, 2020).
- **Reflect on Personal Growth:** Take time to consider how your digital detox has affected other areas of your life. Have you experienced improved focus at work or school? Have your relationships deepened? Acknowledging these broader impacts can help reinforce the value of your efforts (Zario, n.d.).

Sharing Your Experience with Others to Inspire Change

Sharing your journey with others can be a powerful way to inspire change and foster a sense of community. By articulating your experiences and the lessons learned during your digital detox, you can motivate others to reflect on their own technology use and consider making positive changes. Here are some effective ways to share your experience:

- **Social Media:** Use your social media platforms to share your digital detox journey. Post updates about your progress, insights gained, and strategies that worked for you. Consider using relevant hashtags to connect with others who are interested in digital wellness (Kuss & Griffiths, 2017). However, be mindful of your own boundaries when sharing online, as the goal is to promote positive engagement rather than revert to old habits.
- **Blogging or Vlogging:** If you enjoy writing or creating videos, consider starting a blog or vlog to document your digital detox journey. Share your experiences, challenges, and successes, and provide tips for others who may want to embark on a similar path. This can create a supportive community and encourage dialogue about healthy technology use (Davis, 2020).
- **Host a Discussion Group:** Organize a discussion group with friends, family, or colleagues to talk about your experiences and the importance of mindful technology use. This can be an informal gathering or a more structured event, such as a workshop. Sharing your journey in a group setting can foster meaningful conversations and inspire others to reflect on their own digital habits (Zario, n.d.).
- **Engage with Local Organizations:** Reach out to local organizations or community groups focused on mental health, wellness, or technology use. Offer to share your story or facilitate a workshop on digital detox strategies. By engaging with your community, you can inspire others to consider their relationship with technology and promote healthier habits (Kuss & Griffiths, 2017).

Reflecting on your journey through the 30-Day Digital Detox Challenge is an essential step in solidifying the positive changes you've made. By celebrating your progress and achievements, you reinforce your commitment to maintaining healthy digital habits. Additionally, sharing your experiences with others can inspire change and foster a sense of community around mindful technology use. Embrace this opportunity for reflection as a means of growth, connection, and empowerment, and carry the lessons learned into your future digital life.

References

- Davis, J. (2020). The power of reflection: How to celebrate your achievements. Mindful Living. https://www.mindfulliving.com/power-of-reflection-celebrate-your-achievements/

- Kuss, D. J., & Griffiths, M. D. (2017). Social networking sites and addiction: Ten lessons learned. International Journal of Environmental Research and Public Health, 14(3), 311. https://doi.org/10.3390/ijerph14030311
- Zario. (n.d.). Prioritizing digital wellbeing: A guide to mindful technology use. https://www.meetzario.com/post/prioritizing-digital-wellbeing-a-guide-to-mindful-technology-use

Conclusion

As you conclude your 30-Day Digital Detox Challenge, it's essential to reflect on the journey you've undertaken and the lasting benefits you've gained. This challenge has provided you with the tools and insights necessary to foster a healthier relationship with technology, empowering you to reclaim your time, focus, and happiness. In this final section, we will explore the lasting benefits of your digital detox and how to continue your journey toward a healthier digital life.

The Lasting Benefits of the 30-Day Digital Detox Challenge

- **Enhanced Mental Clarity:** One of the most immediate benefits of your digital detox is the improved mental clarity you have experienced. By reducing distractions and minimizing the constant influx of information, you have created space for deeper thinking and creativity. Many participants in digital detox programs report feeling more focused and productive, as they can engage fully in tasks without the interruptions of notifications and social media (Davis, 2020).

- **Improved Emotional Well-Being:** Throughout the detox, you likely noticed a shift in your emotional state. By stepping away from the pressures of social media and the compulsive need to check your devices, you have reduced feelings of anxiety, stress, and comparison. This newfound emotional balance can lead to increased happiness and satisfaction in your daily life (Kuss & Griffiths, 2017).

- **Strengthened Relationships:** By prioritizing face-to-face interactions and engaging in offline activities, you have fostered deeper connections with friends and family. The quality of your relationships is likely to have improved, as you've been more present and attentive during social interactions. This sense of connection is crucial for emotional well-being and can provide a strong support network in times of need (Holt-Lunstad et al., 2010).

- **Increased Awareness of Technology Use:** The detox has equipped you with a heightened awareness of your digital habits. You are now better able to recognize triggers that lead to excessive screen time and can make more intentional choices about how you engage with technology. This awareness is the foundation for maintaining healthy digital habits moving forward (Zario, n.d.).

As you move beyond the 30-Day Digital Detox Challenge, it's essential to continue nurturing the positive changes you've made. Here are some strategies to help you maintain a healthier digital life:

- **Establish Ongoing Digital Boundaries:** Continue to set boundaries around your technology use. This may include designating tech-free times or spaces, limiting screen time, and regularly assessing your digital habits. By maintaining these boundaries, you can ensure that technology remains a tool for enhancing your life rather than a source of distraction or stress (Dwase, 2022).
- **Practice Mindfulness Regularly:** Incorporate mindfulness practices into your daily routine to help you stay grounded and present. Techniques such as meditation, deep breathing, or journaling can support your mental well-being and reinforce the lessons learned during your detox (Davis, 2020).
- **Engage in Offline Activities:** Make a conscious effort to prioritize offline activities that bring you joy and fulfillment. Whether it's pursuing hobbies, spending time in nature, or connecting with loved ones, these activities can help you maintain a balanced lifestyle and reduce reliance on digital devices (Zario, n.d.).
- **Reflect and Adjust:** Regularly reflect on your relationship with technology and make adjustments as needed. Consider scheduling periodic digital detoxes or check-ins to reassess your habits and ensure you are staying true to your goals (Kuss & Griffiths, 2017).
- Share Your Journey: Continue to share your experiences and insights with others. By discussing your journey, you can inspire those around you to consider their own digital habits and promote a culture of mindful technology use (Davis, 2020).

Final Thoughts

The 30-Day Digital Detox Challenge is not just a one-time event; it is the beginning of a lifelong journey toward a healthier digital life. By embracing the benefits of your detox and committing to ongoing mindful technology use, you can create a more balanced and fulfilling existence. Remember that the goal is not to eliminate technology entirely but to cultivate a relationship with it that enhances your life rather than detracts from it. As you move forward, carry the lessons learned and the positive changes made into your everyday life, and enjoy the lasting benefits of a more intentional and mindful approach to technology.

TOOLS

Monthly, Weekly and Daily Digital Detox Challenge

The first 30 - Day Digital Detox Challenge

Day	Focus	Activities
1	Setting Goals	- Reflect on your motivations for the detox - Set specific, achievable goals - Write down your goals and post them in a visible

		place
2	Preparing Your Environment	- Identify tech-free zones in your home (e.g., bedroom, dining area) - Remove devices from these zones and keep them out of sight - Inform friends and family about your digital detox
3	Identifying Triggers	- Reflect on when and why you typically use digital devices - Note down specific triggers (e.g., boredom, stress, FOMO) - Develop strategies to mitigate these triggers
4	Reducing Overall Screen Time	- Gradually reduce your overall screen time by 30 minutes - Set a timer to track your usage and stick to your limit - Engage in an offline activity when the timer goes off
5	Avoiding Devices During Mealtimes	- Keep devices out of sight during mealtimes - Engage in conversation with family or friends - Savor your food and be present in the moment
6	Engaging in Offline Activities	- Spend at least 30 minutes engaged in an offline hobby or activity - Read a book, write in a journal, or work on a craft project - Avoid using devices during this time
7	Preparing for a Tech-Free Weekend	- Gradually reduce your overall screen time by an additional 30 minutes - Plan offline activities and outings for the upcoming weekend - Inform friends and family about your tech-free weekend

8	Mindful Social Media Use	- Limit social media usage to 30 minutes per day - Be intentional about what you post and engage with - Unfollow accounts that trigger negative emotions or comparisons
9	Avoiding Devices 1 Hour Before Bed	- Avoid using devices for 1 hour before your scheduled bedtime - Engage in relaxing activities like reading, stretching, or meditation - Prioritize getting enough sleep
10	Reflecting on the First Week	- Review your progress and celebrate your achievements so far - Reflect on the lessons learned and insights gained - Adjust your goals or strategies if needed
11	Spending Time in Nature	- Spend at least 30 minutes outdoors, either in your backyard or a local park - Engage in a nature-based activity like birdwatching, gardening, or a short hike - Observe and appreciate your surroundings with all your senses
12	Connecting with Friends Offline	- Schedule an in-person meetup with a friend or family member - Engage in a tech-free activity like going for a walk, cooking together, or playing a board game - Practice active listening and being present during the interaction
13	Engaging in Outdoor Activities	- Plan an outdoor adventure, such as a picnic, a bike ride, or a visit to a local attraction - Invite friends or family members to join you - Capture memories through photos or sketches instead of posting on social media

14	Reflecting on the Second Week	- Review your progress and celebrate your achievements so far - Reflect on the lessons learned and insights gained - Adjust your goals or strategies if needed
15	Digital Detox Weekend Begins	- Completely abstain from using digital devices for the next 48 hours - Engage in offline activities and hobbies - Spend quality time with loved ones
16	Digital Detox Weekend Continues	- Continue to abstain from using digital devices - Engage in relaxing activities like reading, crafting, or playing games - Spend time in nature or participate in outdoor activities
17	Digital Detox Weekend Ends	- Gradually reintroduce digital devices into your routine - Reflect on your experiences and insights gained during the detox - Share your thoughts with friends and family
18	Mindful Work Habits	- Set boundaries around work-related technology use - Avoid checking emails or Slack messages outside of work hours - Take regular breaks from screens to stretch, meditate, or engage in offline tasks
19	Cultivating Healthy Sleep Habits	- Establish a consistent sleep routine by going to bed and waking up at the same time each day - Avoid using devices for 1 hour before your scheduled bedtime - Create a relaxing bedtime routine to help you wind down

20	Incorporating Physical Activity	- Engage in at least 30 minutes of physical activity, such as walking, yoga, or a workout video - Find an activity you enjoy and make it a part of your daily routine - Avoid using devices during your workout
21	Reflecting on the Third Week	- Review your progress and celebrate your achievements so far - Reflect on the lessons learned and insights gained - Adjust your goals or strategies if needed
22	Practicing Mindfulness	- Set aside 10-15 minutes each day for mindfulness practice - Try different techniques like meditation, deep breathing, or body scans - Notice how mindfulness affects your mood and focus throughout the day
23	Engaging in Creative Pursuits	- Spend at least 30 minutes engaged in a creative activity, such as writing, painting, or playing a musical instrument - Allow yourself to be fully immersed in the creative process - Avoid using devices during this time
24	Reflecting on the Fourth Week	- Review your progress and celebrate your achievements so far - Reflect on the lessons learned and insights gained - Adjust your goals or strategies if needed
25	Planning for the Future	- Reflect on your experiences during the digital detox - Identify the habits and strategies that worked best for you - Develop a plan for maintaining healthy digital habits moving forward

26	Sharing Your Experience	- Write a blog post, create a video, or share your story on social media - Inspire others by sharing the benefits of your digital detox - Encourage friends and family to join you in cultivating healthier digital habits
27	Celebrating Your Achievements	- Reflect on your progress and celebrate your achievements - Treat yourself to something special, such as a favorite meal or activity - Recognize how far you've come and the positive changes you've made
28	Reintroducing Technology Mindfully	- Gradually reintroduce digital devices into your routine - Be intentional about how and why you use technology - Set boundaries and limits to maintain a healthy balance
29	Continuing Your Journey	- Reflect on the lessons learned and insights gained during the detox - Identify ways to incorporate these lessons into your daily life - Commit to maintaining healthy digital habits moving forward
30	Celebrating the End of the Challenge	- Reflect on your overall experience and the benefits you've gained - Celebrate your commitment and the positive changes you've made - Share your experience with others to inspire change

The Second 30 - Day Digital Detox Challenge

Day	Challenge
1	Turn off all notifications (social media, emails, apps).
2	Set a daily screen time limit (e.g., 2 hours max for non-work-related use).
3	Designate phone-free zones (e.g., bedroom, dining table).
4	Use grayscale mode on your phone to reduce its appeal.
5	Unfollow/unsubscribe from unnecessary social media accounts and emails.
6	Limit yourself to checking social media once in the morning and once in the evening.
7	No social media for the entire day.
8	Spend 1 hour outdoors without your phone.
9	Declutter your apps – delete those you haven't used in 30 days.
10	Create a morning routine without checking your phone for the first hour after waking up.
11	No phone during meals for the entire day.
12	Set an auto-reply for emails and avoid checking them outside work hours.
13	Use your phone only for calls and texts today (no social media or apps).
14	Have a phone-free evening after 7 PM.
15	No digital entertainment (TV, streaming, video games) for the day.
16	Delete one social media app you find addictive (temporarily or permanently).
17	Replace 1 hour of screen time with a new hobby (reading, exercising, etc.).
18	Schedule a 30-minute "tech-free" break during work hours.
19	Go for a walk without your phone and focus on being mindful of your surroundings.
20	Avoid using your phone for the first 2 hours after waking up.
21	Have a completely screen-free day (no phones, TV, computers, or tablets).
22	Limit social media use to 30 minutes for the day.
23	Do not check your phone while commuting.
24	Practice a 10-minute mindfulness meditation without any gadgets.
25	Write in a journal instead of using your phone before bed.
26	Watch a sunset or sunrise without any digital distractions.
27	Set up an evening wind-down routine, avoiding screens 1 hour before bed.
28	Spend an afternoon with friends or family, leaving your phone at home or in airplane mode.

| 29 | No digital devices after 8 PM for the entire day. |
| 30 | Reflect on your 30-day detox journey and set long-term goals for maintaining a healthy digital diet. |

MUSLIMS 30 - Day Digital Detox Challenge

Day	Focus	Activities
1	Intention	- Set a sincere intention (niyyah) for the detox. - Reflect on the importance of reducing distractions to

	Setting	reconnect with your faith.
2	Assess Digital Habits	- Evaluate your current digital usage. - Identify apps or activities that distract you from your spiritual goals.
3	Goal Setting	- Set specific, achievable goals for your digital detox (e.g., reduce social media time, limit news consumption). - Write down your goals and keep them visible.
4	Gradual Reduction	- Reduce screen time by 30 minutes today. - Use that time for extra prayers or reading the Quran.
5	Morning Routine	- Avoid using devices for the first hour after waking up. - Spend this time in dhikr, du'a, and reflection.
6	Evening Routine	- Avoid using devices for the last hour before bed. - Engage in reading or journaling about your day.
7	Tech-Free Zones	- Designate specific areas in your home as tech-free zones (e.g., prayer room, dining area). - Keep devices out of these spaces.
8	Mindful Social Media Use	- Limit social media usage to 30 minutes today. - Be intentional about what you post and engage with.
9	Notification Management	- Unsubscribe from non-essential notifications and emails. - Focus on digital interactions that support your spiritual growth.
10	Reflection	- Reflect on your progress so far. - Journal about your experiences and insights gained during the detox.

11	Connecting with Nature	- Spend time outdoors for at least 30 minutes. - Engage in a nature-based activity while reflecting on Allah's creation.
12	Face-to-Face Interactions	- Schedule an in-person meetup with a friend or family member. - Engage in a tech-free activity together, such as a walk or meal.
13	Community Engagement	- Attend a local Islamic event or class. - Engage with your community and deepen your connections.
14	Volunteering	- Volunteer your time to help with community activities (e.g., iftar preparations, teaching). - Focus on giving back to your community.
15	Digital Detox Weekend	- Completely abstain from using digital devices for the next 48 hours. - Use this time for prayer, reading, and spending quality time with family.
16	Digital Detox Weekend Continues	- Continue to engage in offline activities. - Reflect on your experiences during the detox.
17	Digital Detox Weekend Ends	- Gradually reintroduce digital devices into your routine. - Reflect on the benefits you experienced during the detox.
18	Mindful Work Habits	- Set boundaries around work-related technology use. - Avoid checking emails or work messages outside of work hours.

19	Healthy Sleep Habits	- Establish a consistent sleep routine by going to bed and waking up at the same time. - Avoid screens before bedtime to improve sleep quality.
20	Incorporating Physical Activity	- Engage in at least 30 minutes of physical activity (e.g., walking, jogging, or yoga). - Avoid using devices during your workout.
21	Reflection	- Review your progress and celebrate your achievements. - Reflect on the lessons learned and insights gained.
22	Practicing Mindfulness	- Set aside 10-15 minutes each day for mindfulness practice (e.g., meditation, deep breathing). - Notice how mindfulness affects your mood and focus.
23	Engaging in Creative Pursuits	- Spend at least 30 minutes engaged in a creative activity (e.g., writing, painting). - Allow yourself to be fully immersed in the creative process.
24	Reflection	- Reflect on your overall experience during the digital detox. - Journal about your growth and changes in your digital habits.
25	Planning for the Future	- Identify the habits and strategies that worked best for you. - Develop a plan for maintaining healthy digital habits moving forward.
26	Sharing Your Experience	- Write a blog post or share your story on social media. - Inspire others by discussing the benefits of your digital detox.
27	Celebrating	- Reflect on your progress and celebrate your achievements. - Treat yourself to something special as a reward for your

	Achievements	commitment.
28	Reintroducing Technology Mindfully	- Gradually reintroduce digital devices into your routine. - Be intentional about how and why you use technology.
29	Continuing Your Journey	- Reflect on the lessons learned during the detox. - Commit to maintaining healthy digital habits moving forward.
30	Final Reflection	- Celebrate the completion of your digital detox. - Share your experience with others to inspire change and promote mindfulness in technology use.

CHRISTIANS 30 - Day Digital Detox Challenge for Christians

Day	Focus	Activities
1	Intention Setting	- Set an intention to draw closer to God through this digital detox. - Pray for God's guidance and strength throughout the process.
2	Assessing Digital Habits	- Evaluate your current digital usage and identify areas for improvement. - Notice how technology affects your spiritual life and relationships.
3	Goal Setting	- Prayerfully set specific, achievable goals for your digital detox (e.g., more time in prayer, less social media use). - Write down your goals and keep them visible as a reminder.

4	Gradual Reduction	- Reduce screen time by 30 minutes today. - Use that time for extra prayer, Bible reading, or journaling.
5	Morning Routine	- Begin your day with prayer and Bible reading before using any devices. - Meditate on a verse or passage that will guide your day.
6	Evening Routine	- End your day with prayer, reflection, and gratitude. - Avoid using devices for the last hour before bed.
7	Tech-Free Zones	- Designate specific areas in your home as tech-free zones (e.g., prayer room, dining area). - Keep devices out of these spaces to create a sense of sanctity.
8	Mindful Social Media Use	- Limit social media usage to 30 minutes today. - Be intentional about what you post and engage with, considering how it aligns with your faith.
9	Notification Management	- Unsubscribe from non-essential notifications and emails. - Focus on digital interactions that support your spiritual growth.
10	Reflection	- Reflect on your progress so far through journaling or prayer. - Ask God to reveal any areas where you need to make adjustments.
11	Connecting with Nature	- Spend time outdoors for at least 30 minutes. - Engage in a nature-based activity while reflecting on God's creation.

12	Face-to-Face Interactions	- Schedule an in-person meetup with a Christian friend or family member. - Engage in a tech-free activity together, such as a walk or meal.
13	Community Engagement	- Attend a church event or small group meeting. - Engage with your Christian community and deepen your connections.
14	Serving Others	- Look for opportunities to serve others in your community. - Focus on giving back and sharing God's love without the use of technology.
15	Digital Detox Weekend	- Completely abstain from using digital devices for the next 48 hours. - Use this time for prayer, Bible reading, and spending quality time with family.
16	Digital Detox Weekend Continues	- Continue to engage in offline activities and spiritual practices. - Reflect on your experiences during the detox through journaling or prayer.
17	Digital Detox Weekend Ends	- Gradually reintroduce digital devices into your routine. - Reflect on the benefits you experienced during the detox and how you can maintain healthy habits.
18	Mindful Work Habits	- Set boundaries around work-related technology use. - Avoid checking emails or work messages outside of work hours.
19	Healthy Sleep Habits	- Establish a consistent sleep routine by going to

		bed and waking up at the same time. - Avoid screens before bedtime to improve sleep quality and allow for more time in prayer.
20	Incorporating Physical Activity	- Engage in at least 30 minutes of physical activity (e.g., walking, jogging, or yoga). - Use this time to pray, listen to Christian music, or meditate on Scripture.
21	Reflection	- Review your progress and celebrate your achievements. - Reflect on the lessons learned and insights gained through prayer and journaling.
22	Practicing Mindfulness	- Set aside 10-15 minutes each day for mindfulness practice (e.g., meditation, deep breathing). - Focus on being present with God and allowing Him to speak to your heart.
23	Engaging in Creative Pursuits	- Spend at least 30 minutes engaged in a creative activity (e.g., writing, painting, crafting). - Allow yourself to be fully immersed in the creative process while considering how it glorifies God.
24	Reflection	- Reflect on your overall experience during the digital detox through prayer and journaling. - Ask God to reveal any areas where you need to make lasting changes.
25	Planning for the Future	- Identify the habits and strategies that worked best for you. - Develop a plan for maintaining healthy digital habits moving forward, grounded in your faith.

26	Sharing Your Experience	- Write a blog post or share your story on social media. - Inspire others by discussing the spiritual benefits of your digital detox.
27	Celebrating Achievements	- Reflect on your progress and celebrate your achievements through prayer and thanksgiving. - Treat yourself to something special as a reward for your commitment.
28	Reintroducing Technology Mindfully	- Gradually reintroduce digital devices into your routine. - Be intentional about how and why you use technology, keeping God at the center.
29	Continuing Your Journey	- Reflect on the lessons learned during the detox and how you can apply them to your daily life. - Commit to maintaining healthy digital habits moving forward, relying on God's strength.
30	Final Reflection	- Celebrate the completion of your digital detox through prayer and thanksgiving. - Share your experience with others to inspire change and promote mindfulness in technology use, always pointing back to God's glory.

Students 30 - Day Digital Detox Challenge

Day	Focus	Activities
1	Intention Setting	- Set clear intentions for your digital detox. - Reflect on how reducing screen time can help you achieve your academic and personal goals.
2	Assessing Digital Habits	- Track your digital usage for the day to understand how much time you spend on devices. - Identify apps or activities that distract you from studying or self-care.
3	Goal Setting	- Set specific, achievable goals for your digital detox (e.g., reduce social media use, limit gaming). - Write down your goals and keep them visible as a reminder.
4	Gradual Reduction	- Reduce overall screen time by 30 minutes today. - Use that time for studying, reading, or engaging in a hobby.
5	Morning Routine	- Start your day without checking devices for the first hour. - Use this time for breakfast, prayer, or planning your day.
6	Evening Routine	- Avoid using devices for the last hour before bed. - Engage in relaxing activities like reading or journaling.

7	Tech-Free Study Zones	- Designate specific areas in your study space as tech-free zones. - Keep devices out of these spaces to create a focused environment.
8	Mindful Social Media Use	- Limit social media usage to 30 minutes today. - Be intentional about what you post and engage with.
9	Notification Management	- Turn off non-essential notifications on your devices. - Focus on studying without distractions from alerts.
10	Reflection	- Reflect on your progress so far through journaling. - Consider how your digital habits have changed and what you've learned.
11	Connecting with Nature	- Spend at least 30 minutes outdoors, engaging in a nature-based activity. - Reflect on your surroundings and enjoy the fresh air.
12	Face-to-Face Interactions	- Schedule an in-person meetup with a friend or classmate. - Engage in a tech-free activity together, such as studying or having a meal.
13	Community Engagement	- Participate in a school or community event. - Engage with peers and deepen your connections.
14	Volunteering	- Volunteer your time for a local organization or school activity. - Focus on giving back and making a positive

		impact.
15	Digital Detox Weekend	- Completely abstain from using digital devices for the next 48 hours. - Use this time for studying, hobbies, and spending quality time with family and friends.
16	Digital Detox Weekend Continues	- Continue to engage in offline activities and reflect on your experiences during the detox. - Journal about what you enjoyed during your tech-free time.
17	Digital Detox Weekend Ends	- Gradually reintroduce digital devices into your routine. - Reflect on the benefits you experienced during the detox.
18	Mindful Study Habits	- Set boundaries around study-related technology use. - Avoid checking social media or personal messages while studying.
19	Healthy Sleep Habits	- Establish a consistent sleep routine by going to bed and waking up at the same time. - Avoid screens before bedtime to improve sleep quality.
20	Incorporating Physical Activity	- Engage in at least 30 minutes of physical activity (e.g., walking, jogging, or yoga). - Use this time to clear your mind and recharge.
21	Reflection	- Review your progress and celebrate your achievements. - Reflect on the lessons learned and insights gained through journaling.

22	Practicing Mindfulness	- Set aside 10-15 minutes each day for mindfulness practice (e.g., meditation, deep breathing). - Focus on being present and aware of your thoughts and feelings.
23	Engaging in Creative Pursuits	- Spend at least 30 minutes engaged in a creative activity (e.g., drawing, writing, or crafting). - Allow yourself to be fully immersed in the creative process.
24	Reflection	- Reflect on your overall experience during the digital detox. - Journal about your growth and changes in your digital habits.
25	Planning for the Future	- Identify the habits and strategies that worked best for you. - Develop a plan for maintaining healthy digital habits moving forward.
26	Sharing Your Experience	- Share your detox journey with friends or classmates. - Inspire others by discussing the benefits of your digital detox.
27	Celebrating Achievements	- Reflect on your progress and celebrate your achievements. - Treat yourself to something special as a reward for your commitment.
28	Reintroducing Technology Mindfully	- Gradually reintroduce digital devices into your routine. - Be intentional about how and why you use technology, focusing on academic and personal

Day	Focus	Activities
		growth.
29	Continuing Your Journey	- Reflect on the lessons learned during the detox and how you can apply them to your daily life. - Commit to maintaining healthy digital habits moving forward.
30	Final Reflection	- Celebrate the completion of your digital detox. - Share your experience with others to inspire change and promote mindfulness in technology use.

Chief Executive Officer (CEO) 30 - Day Digital Detox Challenge

Day	Focus	Activities
1	Intention Setting	- Reflect on your motivations for the detox. - Set specific goals (e.g., reduce screen time, improve sleep, enhance focus).
2	Assess Digital Habits	- Track your digital usage for a day to identify patterns. - Note which apps and activities consume the most time.
3	Goal Setting	- Define clear, measurable goals for your detox (e.g., limit social media to 15 minutes per day). - Write down your goals and share them with a

		trusted colleague for accountability.
4	Notification Management	- Turn off non-essential notifications on your devices. - Set specific times for checking emails and messages.
5	Tech-Free Mornings	- Commit to not checking your phone for the first hour after waking up. - Use this time for exercise, meditation, or planning your day.
6	Evening Routine	- Avoid using devices for the last hour before bed. - Engage in relaxing activities such as reading or journaling.
7	Digital-Free Zones	- Designate specific areas in your home or office as tech-free zones (e.g., dining table, bedroom). - Enjoy device-free meals and conversations.
8	Social Media Detox	- Limit social media usage to 15 minutes today. - Reflect on how this impacts your mood and productivity.
9	Digital Declutter	- Unsubscribe from unnecessary emails and notifications. - Organize your digital workspace (emails, files) to reduce clutter.
10	Reflection	- Reflect on your progress so far and journal about your experiences. - Assess how your digital habits have changed.
11	Connecting with Nature	- Spend at least 30 minutes outdoors today. - Use this time to think creatively or meditate.

12	Face-to-Face Interactions	- Schedule an in-person meeting or lunch with a colleague. - Focus on building relationships without digital distractions.
13	Community Engagement	- Participate in a local business event or networking opportunity. - Engage with peers and deepen your connections.
14	Volunteering	- Dedicate time to volunteer for a cause you care about. - Focus on giving back and making a positive impact.
15	Digital Detox Weekend	- Completely abstain from using digital devices for the next 48 hours. - Use this time for personal reflection, hobbies, and family activities.
16	Digital Detox Weekend Continues	- Continue engaging in offline activities and reflect on your experiences during the detox. - Journal about what you enjoyed during your tech-free time.
17	Digital Detox Weekend Ends	- Gradually reintroduce digital devices into your routine. - Reflect on the benefits you experienced during the detox.
18	Mindful Work Habits	- Set boundaries around work-related technology use. - Avoid checking emails or work messages outside of designated hours.
19	Healthy Sleep Habits	- Establish a consistent sleep routine by going to

		bed and waking up at the same time. - Avoid screens before bedtime to improve sleep quality.
20	Incorporating Physical Activity	- Engage in at least 30 minutes of physical activity (e.g., walking, jogging). - Use this time to clear your mind and recharge.
21	Reflection	- Review your progress and celebrate your achievements. - Reflect on the lessons learned and insights gained through journaling.
22	Practicing Mindfulness	- Set aside 10-15 minutes each day for mindfulness practice (e.g., meditation, deep breathing). - Focus on being present and aware of your thoughts and feelings.
23	Engaging in Creative Pursuits	- Spend at least 30 minutes engaged in a creative activity (e.g., brainstorming, writing). - Allow yourself to be fully immersed in the creative process.
24	Reflection	- Reflect on your overall experience during the digital detox. - Journal about your growth and changes in your digital habits.
25	Planning for the Future	- Identify the habits and strategies that worked best for you. - Develop a plan for maintaining healthy digital habits moving forward.
26	Sharing Your	- Share your detox journey with colleagues or peers.

	Experience	- Inspire others by discussing the benefits of your digital detox.
27	Celebrating Achievements	- Reflect on your progress and celebrate your achievements. - Treat yourself to something special as a reward for your commitment.
28	Reintroducing Technology Mindfully	- Gradually reintroduce digital devices into your routine. - Be intentional about how and why you use technology, focusing on productivity and personal well-being.
29	Continuing Your Journey	- Reflect on the lessons learned during the detox and how you can apply them to your daily life. - Commit to maintaining healthy digital habits moving forward.
30	Final Reflection	- Celebrate the completion of your digital detox. - Share your experience with others to inspire change and promote mindfulness in technology use.

Daily Digital Detox Scheduler

Time	SUNDAY	MONDAY	TUESDAY	WEDNESDAY	THURSDAY	FRIDAY	SATURDAY
6:00 AM							
6:20 AM							
6:40 AM							
7:00 AM							
7:20 AM							
7:40 AM							
8:00 AM							
8:20 AM							
8:40 AM							
9:00 AM							
9:20 AM							
9:40 AM							
10:00 AM							
10:20 AM							
10:40 AM							
11:00 AM							
11:20 AM							
11:40 AM							
12:00 PM							
12:20 PM							
12:40 PM							
1:00 PM							
1:20 PM							
1:40 PM							
2:00 PM							
2:20 PM							
2:40 PM							
3:00 PM							
3:20 PM							
3:40 PM							
4:00 PM							
4:20 PM							
4:40 PM							
5:00 PM							
5:20 PM							
5:40 PM							
6:00 PM							
6:20 PM							
6:40 PM							
7:00 PM							
7:20 PM							
7:40 PM							
8:00 PM							
8:20 PM							
8:40 PM							
9:00 PM							
9:20 PM							
9:40 PM							
10:00 PM							
10:20 PM							
10:40 PM							

Time							
11:00 PM							
11:20 PM							
11:40 PM							
12:00 AM							

Example of a Daily Digital Detox Scheduler

Time	SUNDAY	MONDAY	TUESDAY	WEDNESDAY	THURSDAY	FRIDAY	SATURDAY
6:00 AM	Morning stretch and yoga	Morning walk	Morning stretch and yoga	Meditation	Morning walk	Morning stretch	Yoga
6:20 AM	Morning walk outdoors	Breakfast prep	Journaling	Stretching	Journaling	Meditation	Stretching
6:40 AM	Gratitude journaling	Morning exercise	Nature walk	Breakfast prep	Morning walk	Gratitude journaling	Morning walk
7:00 AM	Prepare healthy breakfast	Journaling	Reading	Morning walk	Reading	Prepare breakfast	Reading
7:20 AM	Breakfast	Stretching	Meditation	Breakfast	Breakfast	Stretching	Breakfast
7:40 AM	Mindful breakfast	Planning the day	Planning the day	Journaling	Planning the day	Mindful breakfast	Planning the day
8:00 AM	Read a book	Read a book	Outdoor exercise	Read a book	Read a book	Outdoor exercise	Meditation
8:20 AM	Go for a nature walk	Write in journal	Yoga practice	Write in journal	Write in journal	Meditation	Journaling
8:40 AM	Journal thoughts	Yoga	Write in journal	Yoga	Outdoor exercise	Write in journal	Yoga
9:00 AM	Work on a creative hobby	Declutter space	Declutter workspace	Work on a creative hobby	Declutter home	Work on a hobby	Declutter space
9:20 AM	Declutter home	Mindful tea break	Gardening	Gardening	Mindful tea break	Gardening	Mindful tea break
9:40 AM	Meditate for 10 minutes	Nature walk	Declutter workspace	Mindful tea break	Nature walk	Declutter workspace	Nature walk
10:00 AM	Gardening	Creative writing	Mindful activity	Creative writing	Gardening	Mindful activity	Gardening
10:20 AM	Water the plants	Mindful journaling	Prepare healthy snack	Journal gratitude	Outdoor activity	Prepare healthy snack	Journal gratitude
10:40 AM	Play a board game	Prepare snack	Read a book	Play a board game	Creative writing	Read a book	Play a board game
11:00 AM	Reading	Visit a local park	Go for a walk	Visit a local park	Go for a walk	Mindful activity	Visit a local park
11:20 AM	Outdoor walking	Outdoor walking	Gardening	Gardening	Outdoor walking	Gardening	Outdoor walking
11:40 AM	Write a letter to a friend	Journaling	Play a board game	Write in journal	Play a board game	Write a letter	Write in journal
12:00 PM	Prepare a healthy lunch	Prepare lunch	Mindful lunch	Prepare lunch	Mindful lunch	Prepare lunch	Mindful lunch
12:20 PM	Mindful lunch	Reflect on your goals	Creative writing	Reflect on your goals	Reflect on goals	Creative writing	Reflect on your goals
12:40 PM	Reading	Light stretching	Reading	Light stretching	Stretching	Reading	Light stretching
1:00 PM	Plan the week	Journaling	Plan for the week	Journaling	Plan for the week	Journaling	Plan for the week
1:20 PM	Nature walk	Meditation	Water the plants	Meditation	Gardening	Meditation	Water the plants
1:40 PM	Listen to nature sounds	Play music	Outdoor walk	Play music	Listen to nature sounds	Outdoor walk	Play music
2:00 PM	Practice a new hobby	Work on hobby	Drawing or painting	Work on hobby	Drawing	Painting	Work on hobby
2:20 PM	Painting or drawing	Organize workspace	Organize workspace	Painting or drawing	Organize workspace	Organize workspace	Painting or drawing
2:40 PM	Visit a local park	Visit a friend	Reflect on the day	Visit a local park	Visit a friend	Reflect on the day	Visit a local park
3:00	Play a board	Play sports	Gardening	Play a board	Play sports	Gardening	Play a board

	SUNDAY	MONDAY	TUESDAY	WEDNESDAY	THURSDAY	FRIDAY	SATURDAY
PM	game			game			game
3:20 PM	Gardening	Take a walk	Mindful meditation	Take a walk	Take a walk	Mindful meditation	Take a walk
3:40 PM	Write in journal	Write letters	Creative writing	Write in journal	Write letters	Creative writing	Write in journal
4:00 PM	Prepare a healthy snack	Tea with family	Tea with family	Prepare a healthy snack	Tea with family	Prepare a healthy snack	Tea with family
4:20 PM	Tea break	Quiet time with a book	Journaling	Tea break	Quiet time with a book	Journaling	Tea break
4:40 PM	Stretch	Play sports	Gardening	Stretch	Play sports	Gardening	Stretch
5:00 PM	Prepare dinner	Listen to relaxing music	Meditate for 10 minutes	Listen to relaxing music	Meditate for 10 minutes	Listen to relaxing music	Meditate for 10 minutes
5:20 PM	Play music	Read a book	Write a gratitude list	Read a book	Write a gratitude list	Read a book	Write a gratitude list
5:40 PM	Quiet reflection	Prepare dinner	Quiet reflection	Prepare dinner	Quiet reflection	Prepare dinner	Quiet reflection
6:00 PM	Prepare dinner	Mindful walk	Play sports	Mindful walk	Play sports	Mindful walk	Play sports
6:20 PM	Family time	Quiet reflection	Tea break	Quiet reflection	Family time	Tea break	Family time
6:40 PM	Dinner with family	Dinner with family	Dinner with family	Dinner with family	Dinner with family	Dinner with family	Dinner with family
7:00 PM	Evening walk	Evening walk	Relaxation	Evening walk	Relaxation	Evening walk	Relaxation
7:20 PM	Play music	Play board games	Yoga session	Play music	Play board games	Yoga session	Play music
7:40 PM	Reading	Reading	Reflect on the day	Reading	Reflect on the day	Reading	Reflect on the day
8:00 PM	Evening wind down	Evening wind down	Mindful meditation	Evening wind down	Evening wind down	Mindful meditation	Evening wind down
8:20 PM	Journaling	Meditation	Journaling	Meditation	Journaling	Meditation	Journaling
8:40 PM	Read a book	Write in gratitude journal	Read a book	Write in gratitude journal	Read a book	Write in gratitude journal	Read a book
9:00 PM	Meditation	Sleep routine	Sleep routine	Meditation	Sleep routine	Sleep routine	Meditation
9:20 PM	Relaxation	Lights off	Relaxation	Lights off	Relaxation	Lights off	Relaxation
9:40 PM	Sleep	Sleep	Sleep	Sleep	Sleep	Sleep	Sleep

Example for a Muslim Woman - Daily Digital Detox Scheduler

Time	SUNDAY	MONDAY	TUESDAY	WEDNESDAY	THURSDAY	FRIDAY	SATURDAY
5:00 AM	Fajr prayer and Du'a	Fajr prayer and Du'a	Fajr prayer and Du'a	Fajr prayer and Du'a	Fajr prayer and Du'a	Fajr prayer and Du'a	Fajr prayer and Du'a

Time							
5:20 AM	Qur'an recitation	Qur'an recitation	Qur'an recitation	Qur'an recitation	Qur'an recitation	Qur'an recitation	Qur'an recitation
5:40 AM	Morning dhikr	Morning dhikr	Morning dhikr	Morning dhikr	Morning dhikr	Morning dhikr	Morning dhikr
6:00 AM	Morning walk	Morning exercise	Morning walk	Morning exercise	Morning walk	Morning walk	Morning walk
6:20 AM	Reflection on Islamic teachings	Prepare breakfast	Journaling	Prepare breakfast	Journaling	Prepare breakfast	Journaling
6:40 AM	Prepare breakfast	Reflect on goals	Prepare breakfast	Reflect on goals	Prepare breakfast	Reflect on goals	Prepare breakfast
7:00 AM	Healthy breakfast	Read a book	Healthy breakfast	Read a book	Healthy breakfast	Read a book	Healthy breakfast
7:20 AM	Help with family chores	Yoga/stretching	Family chores	Yoga/stretching	Family chores	Yoga/stretching	Help with family chores
7:40 AM	Read a book	Reflect on the day	Read a book	Reflect on the day	Read a book	Reflect on the day	Read a book
8:00 AM	Islamic lecture online or podcast	Help family with tasks	Help family with tasks	Islamic podcast	Help family with tasks	Help family with tasks	Islamic lecture or podcast
8:20 AM	Islamic study	Plan activities for the day	Islamic study	Plan activities for the day	Islamic study	Plan activities for the day	Islamic study
8:40 AM	Morning exercise	Mindful tea break	Morning exercise	Mindful tea break	Morning exercise	Mindful tea break	Morning exercise
9:00 AM	Creative writing	Gardening	Gardening	Creative writing	Gardening	Gardening	Creative writing
9:20 AM	Organize room	Call family or friends	Organize room	Call family or friends	Organize room	Call family or friends	Organize room
9:40 AM	Qur'an study	Qur'an study	Qur'an study	Qur'an study	Qur'an study	Qur'an study	Qur'an study
10:00 AM	Mid-morning snack	Qur'an memorization	Mid-morning snack	Qur'an memorization	Mid-morning snack	Qur'an memorization	Mid-morning snack
10:20 AM	Reflect on hadith	Reflect on hadith	Reflect on hadith	Reflect on hadith	Reflect on hadith	Reflect on hadith	Reflect on hadith
10:40 AM	Read a book	Outdoor walk	Read a book	Outdoor walk	Read a book	Outdoor walk	Read a book
11:00 AM	Help family with tasks	Help family with tasks	Help family with tasks	Help family with tasks	Help family with tasks	Help family with tasks	Help family with tasks
11:20 AM	Dhikr or Du'a	Dhikr or Du'a	Dhikr or Du'a	Dhikr or Du'a	Dhikr or Du'a	Dhikr or Du'a	Dhikr or Du'a
11:40 AM	Read a book or Islamic literature	Prepare for Dhuhr	Read a book	Prepare for Dhuhr	Read a book	Prepare for Dhuhr	Read a book
12:00 PM	Dhuhr prayer	Dhuhr prayer	Dhuhr prayer	Dhuhr prayer	Dhuhr prayer	Dhuhr prayer	Dhuhr prayer
12:20 PM	Lunch prep	Lunch with family	Lunch prep	Lunch with family	Lunch prep	Lunch with family	Lunch prep
12:40 PM	Lunch with family	Read Qur'an	Lunch with family	Read Qur'an	Lunch with family	Read Qur'an	Lunch with family
1:00 PM	Help clean up after lunch	Reflect on Islamic teachings	Help clean up after lunch	Reflect on Islamic teachings	Help clean up after lunch	Reflect on Islamic teachings	Help clean up after lunch
1:20 PM	Read a book	Dhikr	Read a book	Dhikr	Read a book	Dhikr	Read a book
1:40 PM	Gardening	Family activity	Gardening	Family activity	Gardening	Family activity	Gardening
2:00 PM	Help siblings with homework	Journaling	Help siblings with homework	Journaling	Help siblings with homework	Journaling	Help siblings with homework
2:20 PM	Creative activity (drawing, writing)	Dhikr	Creative activity	Dhikr	Creative activity	Dhikr	Creative activity
2:40 PM	Rest or light stretching	Help with housework	Rest or light stretching	Help with housework	Rest or light stretching	Help with housework	Rest or light stretching
3:00 PM	Read hadith or Islamic books	Islamic study	Read hadith	Islamic study	Read hadith	Islamic study	Read hadith
3:20 PM	Asr prayer	Asr prayer	Asr prayer	Asr prayer	Asr prayer	Asr prayer	Asr prayer
3:40 PM	Light walk or exercise	Spend time with family	Light walk	Spend time with family	Light walk	Spend time with family	Light walk
4:00 PM	Reflect on Islamic goals	Tea with family	Reflect on Islamic goals	Tea with family	Reflect on Islamic goals	Tea with family	Reflect on Islamic goals
4:20	Qur'an study	Journaling	Qur'an study	Journaling	Qur'an study	Journaling	Qur'an study

	SUNDAY	MONDAY	TUESDAY	WEDNESDAY	THURSDAY	FRIDAY	SATURDAY
PM							
4:40 PM	Outdoor time (gardening or walk)	Islamic study	Outdoor time	Islamic study	Outdoor time	Islamic study	Outdoor time
5:00 PM	Help family prepare dinner	Family activity	Help family prepare dinner	Family activity	Help family prepare dinner	Family activity	Help family prepare dinner
5:20 PM	Qur'an memorization	Qur'an recitation	Qur'an memorization	Qur'an recitation	Qur'an memorization	Qur'an recitation	Qur'an memorization
5:40 PM	Tea break	Reflect on the day	Tea break	Reflect on the day	Tea break	Reflect on the day	Tea break
6:00 PM	Maghrib prayer	Maghrib prayer	Maghrib prayer	Maghrib prayer	Maghrib prayer	Maghrib prayer	Maghrib prayer
6:20 PM	Du'a and reflection	Du'a and reflection	Du'a and reflection	Du'a and reflection	Du'a and reflection	Du'a and reflection	Du'a and reflection
6:40 PM	Dinner with family	Dinner with family	Dinner with family	Dinner with family	Dinner with family	Dinner with family	Dinner with family
7:00 PM	Family time	Quiet reflection	Family time	Quiet reflection	Family time	Quiet reflection	Family time
7:20 PM	Dhikr and Du'a	Islamic lecture	Dhikr and Du'a	Islamic lecture	Dhikr and Du'a	Islamic lecture	Dhikr and Du'a
7:40 PM	Reflect on daily accomplishments	Write in journal	Reflect on daily accomplishments	Write in journal	Reflect on daily accomplishments	Write in journal	Reflect on daily accomplishments
8:00 PM	Isha prayer	Isha prayer	Isha prayer	Isha prayer	Isha prayer	Isha prayer	Isha prayer
8:20 PM	Qur'an recitation	Qur'an recitation	Qur'an recitation	Qur'an recitation	Qur'an recitation	Qur'an recitation	Qur'an recitation
8:40 PM	Relax with family	Quiet reflection	Relax with family	Quiet reflection	Relax with family	Quiet reflection	Relax with family
9:00 PM	Write in gratitude journal	Write in gratitude journal	Write in gratitude journal	Write in gratitude journal	Write in gratitude journal	Write in gratitude journal	Write in gratitude journal
9:20 PM	Sleep routine	Sleep routine	Sleep routine	Sleep routine	Sleep routine	Sleep routine	Sleep routine
9:40 PM	Sleep	Sleep	Sleep	Sleep	Sleep	Sleep	Sleep

Example for a Christian Woman - Daily Digital Detox Scheduler

Time	SUNDAY	MONDAY	TUESDAY	WEDNESDAY	THURSDAY	FRIDAY	SATURDAY
6:00 AM	Morning prayer	Morning prayer	Morning prayer	Morning prayer	Morning prayer	Morning prayer	Morning prayer
6:20 AM	Bible reading (Psalms)	Bible reading (Proverbs)	Bible reading (Psalms)	Bible reading (Proverbs)	Bible reading (Psalms)	Bible reading (Proverbs)	Bible reading (Psalms)
6:40 AM	Journaling thoughts	Journaling prayers	Journaling thoughts	Journaling prayers	Journaling thoughts	Journaling prayers	Journaling thoughts
7:00 AM	Morning walk	Stretching exercises	Morning walk	Stretching exercises	Morning walk	Stretching exercises	Morning walk
7:20 AM	Prepare healthy breakfast	Prepare breakfast	Prepare healthy breakfast	Prepare breakfast	Prepare healthy breakfast	Prepare breakfast	Prepare healthy breakfast
7:40	Family	Family	Family	Family breakfast	Family	Family	Family

Time							
AM	breakfast	breakfast	breakfast		breakfast	breakfast	breakfast
8:00 AM	Attend church service	Bible study	Bible study	Bible study	Bible study	Bible study	Bible study
8:20 AM	Church service continues	Reflect on Scripture	Reflect on Scripture	Reflect on Scripture	Reflect on Scripture	Reflect on Scripture	Reflect on Scripture
8:40 AM	Fellowship after church	Outdoor walk	Creative writing	Outdoor walk	Creative writing	Outdoor walk	Creative writing
9:00 AM	Family time	Organize personal space	Organize personal space	Organize personal space	Organize personal space	Organize personal space	Organize personal space
9:20 AM	Quiet reflection	Journaling	Quiet reflection	Journaling	Quiet reflection	Journaling	Quiet reflection
9:40 AM	Call or meet a friend	Family time	Gardening	Family time	Gardening	Family time	Gardening
10:00 AM	Brunch with family	Light stretching	Brunch with family	Light stretching	Brunch with family	Light stretching	Brunch with family
10:20 AM	Bible reading (New Testament)	Bible reading (New Testament)	Bible reading (New Testament)	Bible reading (New Testament)	Bible reading (New Testament)	Bible reading (New Testament)	Bible reading (New Testament)
10:40 AM	Prayer time	Journaling prayers	Prayer time	Journaling prayers	Prayer time	Journaling prayers	Prayer time
11:00 AM	Volunteer or service activity	Outdoor activity	Family service or volunteer work	Outdoor activity	Family service or volunteer work	Outdoor activity	Family service or volunteer work
11:20 AM	Family lunch prep	Lunch prep	Lunch prep	Lunch prep	Lunch prep	Lunch prep	Lunch prep
11:40 AM	Family lunch	Family lunch	Family lunch	Family lunch	Family lunch	Family lunch	Family lunch
12:00 PM	Midday prayer	Quiet reflection	Midday prayer	Quiet reflection	Midday prayer	Quiet reflection	Midday prayer
12:20 PM	Relax with family	Relax with family	Relax with family	Relax with family	Relax with family	Relax with family	Relax with family
12:40 PM	Reflect on morning sermon	Family discussion	Reflect on morning sermon	Family discussion	Reflect on morning sermon	Family discussion	Reflect on morning sermon
1:00 PM	Bible journaling	Journaling prayers	Bible journaling	Journaling prayers	Bible journaling	Journaling prayers	Bible journaling
1:20 PM	Help with chores	Family walk	Help with chores	Family walk	Help with chores	Family walk	Help with chores
1:40 PM	Outdoor activity (gardening, walk)	Quiet time	Outdoor activity (gardening, walk)	Quiet time	Outdoor activity (gardening, walk)	Quiet time	Outdoor activity (gardening, walk)
2:00 PM	Read a Christian book	Call or visit a friend	Read a Christian book	Call or visit a friend	Read a Christian book	Call or visit a friend	Read a Christian book
2:20 PM	Tea or coffee break	Creative writing	Tea or coffee break	Creative writing	Tea or coffee break	Creative writing	Tea or coffee break
2:40 PM	Reflect on Bible verses	Reflect on daily goals	Reflect on Bible verses	Reflect on daily goals	Reflect on Bible verses	Reflect on daily goals	Reflect on Bible verses
3:00 PM	Afternoon prayer	Afternoon prayer	Afternoon prayer	Afternoon prayer	Afternoon prayer	Afternoon prayer	Afternoon prayer
3:20 PM	Rest or light walk	Play music	Rest or light walk	Play music	Rest or light walk	Play music	Rest or light walk
3:40 PM	Read devotional	Journaling	Read devotional	Journaling	Read devotional	Journaling	Read devotional
4:00 PM	Family time	Play games with family	Family time	Play games with family	Family time	Play games with family	Family time
4:20 PM	Plan evening devotion	Organize evening meal	Plan evening devotion	Organize evening meal	Plan evening devotion	Organize evening meal	Plan evening devotion
4:40 PM	Prepare dinner	Evening walk	Prepare dinner	Evening walk	Prepare dinner	Evening walk	Prepare dinner
5:00 PM	Dinner with family	Dinner with family	Dinner with family	Dinner with family	Dinner with family	Dinner with family	Dinner with family
5:20 PM	Evening walk	Bible study	Evening walk	Bible study	Evening walk	Bible study	Evening walk
5:40 PM	Reflect on the day	Reflect on Scripture	Reflect on the day	Reflect on Scripture	Reflect on the day	Reflect on Scripture	Reflect on the day
6:00 PM	Evening prayer	Evening prayer	Evening prayer	Evening prayer	Evening prayer	Evening prayer	Evening prayer

6:20 PM	Quiet reflection	Worship music	Quiet reflection	Worship music	Quiet reflection	Worship music	Quiet reflection
6:40 PM	Bible reading (Old Testament)	Bible reading (Old Testament)	Bible reading (Old Testament)	Bible reading (Old Testament)	Bible reading (Old Testament)	Bible reading (Old Testament)	Bible reading (Old Testament)
7:00 PM	Family game or discussion	Family time	Family game or discussion	Family time	Family game or discussion	Family time	Family game or discussion
7:20 PM	Gratitude journaling	Gratitude journaling	Gratitude journaling	Gratitude journaling	Gratitude journaling	Gratitude journaling	Gratitude journaling
7:40 PM	Listen to worship music	Listen to worship music	Listen to worship music	Listen to worship music	Listen to worship music	Listen to worship music	Listen to worship music
8:00 PM	Evening devotion	Evening devotion	Evening devotion	Evening devotion	Evening devotion	Evening devotion	Evening devotion
8:20 PM	Journaling prayers	Journaling thoughts	Journaling prayers	Journaling thoughts	Journaling prayers	Journaling thoughts	Journaling prayers
8:40 PM	Prepare for bed	Quiet prayer	Prepare for bed	Quiet prayer	Prepare for bed	Quiet prayer	Prepare for bed
9:00 PM	Night prayer	Night prayer	Night prayer	Night prayer	Night prayer	Night prayer	Night prayer
9:20 PM	Bible reading (Psalms)	Bible reading (Psalms)	Bible reading (Psalms)	Bible reading (Psalms)	Bible reading (Psalms)	Bible reading (Psalms)	Bible reading (Psalms)
9:40 PM	Rest and sleep	Rest and sleep	Rest and sleep	Rest and sleep	Rest and sleep	Rest and sleep	Rest and sleep

The 30-Day Digital Detox Challenge by Aliyu Aminu Ahmed

In today's hyper-connected world, we often find ourselves overwhelmed by constant notifications, social media updates, and digital distractions. The 30-Day Digital Detox Challenge offers a practical and transformative guide to help you reclaim your time, focus, and overall well-being.

Author Aliyu Aminu Ahmed presents a step-by-step program that encourages a healthier relationship with technology by helping you reflect on your digital habits and replace screen time with meaningful, enriching activities. This challenge is more than just unplugging—it's about reconnecting with yourself, your loved ones, and the world around you.

Throughout this book, you'll find strategies to reduce screen time, avoid digital overload, and cultivate mindfulness in your daily life. Whether you are a busy professional, student, or anyone seeking balance in a tech-driven world, this 30-day journey offers the tools and support needed for lasting change. With insights on managing digital addiction and practical advice for establishing healthier routines, you'll discover how to regain control of your digital life and embrace a more fulfilling, present lifestyle.

Extra Resources

S/N	Resource	Description	Link
1	Newport, C. (2019). *Digital Minimalism: Choosing a Focused Life in a Noisy World*. Portfolio.	This book explores the philosophy of digital minimalism, advocating for a more intentional approach to technology use. Newport provides practical advice for reducing digital distractions and enhancing focus on what truly matters.	https://www.amazon.com/Digital-Minimalism-Choosing-Focused-Noisy/dp/0525536515
2	Price, C. (2018). *How to Break Up with Your Phone: The 30-Day Plan to Take Back Your Life*. Ten Speed Press.	Price offers a step-by-step guide to reducing phone dependency. The book includes a 30-day plan that helps readers understand their relationship with their devices and develop healthier habits.	https://www.catherineprice.com/how-to-break-up-with-your-phone
3	Carr, N. (2011). *The Shallows: What the Internet Is Doing to*	This thought-provoking book examines how constant internet use	https://wwnorton.com/books/

	Our Brains. W. W. Norton & Company.	affects our cognitive abilities, attention spans, and overall mental health. Carr's insights encourage readers to reconsider their digital habits.	978039335782 0
4	Eyal, N. (2019). *" Indistractable": How to Control Your Attention and Choose Your Life*. BenBella Books.	Eyal provides strategies for maintaining focus and avoiding distractions in a technology-driven world. The book emphasizes the importance of self-awareness and intentionality in technology use.	https://www.in distractable.co m
5	Zahariades, D. (2019). *Digital Detox: The 30-Day Challenge to Reclaim Your Life*. Art of Productivity.	This practical guide offers a comprehensive plan for reducing screen time and improving overall well-being. Zahariades provides actionable steps and tips for maintaining a balanced digital life.	https://www.ar tofproductivity .com/digital-detox
6	Digital Detox Community. (n.d.). Facebook.	This group provides a supportive environment for individuals looking to reduce their screen time and engage in digital detox challenges. Members share experiences, tips, and encouragement.	https://www.fa cebook.com/gr oups/digitaldet oxcommunity
7	Mindful Techie Community. (n.d.). Mindful Techie.	An online community focused on promoting mindfulness in technology use. Members can participate in discussions, share resources, and support one another in their digital wellness journeys.	https://www.m indfultechie.co m
8	Reddit - Digital Minimalism. (n.d.). Reddit.	This subreddit is dedicated to discussions about digital minimalism, providing a space for individuals to share their experiences, challenges, and successes in reducing screen time.	https://www.re ddit.com/r/digi talminimalism
9	Screen Time Support Groups. (n.d.). Facebook.	Various online forums and support groups focus on managing screen time and technology use. These groups often provide resources, advice, and accountability for individuals seeking to make positive changes.	https://www.fa cebook.com/gr oups/screentim esupportgroups
10	Meetup Groups for Mindfulness and Digital Detox. (n.d.). Meetup.	Check local Meetup groups for gatherings focused on mindfulness, meditation, and digital detox. These groups often provide opportunities	https://www.m eetup.com/topi cs/mindfulness -digital-detox

		for in-person support and community engagement.	
11	Forest. (n.d.). Stay focused, be present.	This app encourages users to stay focused by planting virtual trees that grow while they avoid using their phones. If users exit the app, the tree dies, promoting mindfulness and concentration.	https://www.forestapp.cc
12	Freedom. (n.d.). Block distracting websites & apps.	A website and app blocker that allows users to block distracting websites and apps across all devices. Users can customize their blocking schedules to maintain focus during work or study sessions.	https://freedom.to
13	StayFocusd. (n.d.). Stay focused on what matters.	A browser extension that limits the amount of time users can spend on distracting websites. It helps individuals stay productive by encouraging mindful browsing habits.	https://chrome.google.com/webstore/detail/stayfocusd/laankejkbhbdhmipfmgcngdelahlfoji
14	Headspace. (n.d.). Meditation and sleep made simple.	A mindfulness and meditation app that offers guided sessions to help users manage stress, improve focus, and cultivate a sense of calm. It can be a valuable tool for integrating mindfulness into daily routines.	https://www.headspace.com
15	Screen Time (iOS). (n.d.). Apple Support.	Built-in features on iOS devices that track usage patterns and allow users to set limits on app usage. These tools help individuals become more aware of their digital habits.	https://support.apple.com/en-us/HT208982
16	Digital Wellbeing (Android). (n.d.). Google.	Built-in features on Android devices that track usage patterns and allow users to set limits on app usage. These tools help individuals become more aware of their digital habits.	https://wellbeing.google
17	Calm. (n.d.). The #1 app for meditation and sleep.	An app that offers meditation, sleep stories, and relaxation techniques. It provides resources for users to incorporate mindfulness practices into their daily lives.	https://www.calm.com
18	Insight Timer. (n.d.). Free meditation app.	A free meditation app with a large library of guided meditations, music tracks, and talks by mindfulness experts. It helps users cultivate a	https://insighttimer.com

		consistent meditation practice.	